Victory over Pancreatic Cancer

A Survivor's Story of Life, Love, and Faith

by Sarah Burton

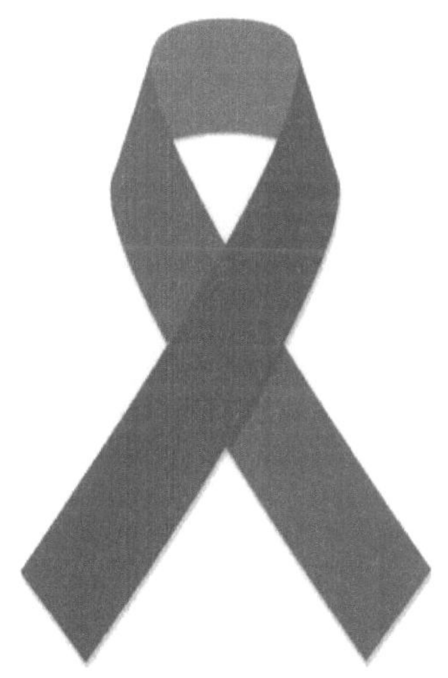

This is a non-fiction memoir and some names are initialed for privacy purposes.

Text copyright © 2019 by Sarah Burton

ISBN 9781712546437
December 2019

This book is dedicated to all of the pancreatic cancer patients and survivors who have suffered this most terrible and lethal disease.

I want this book to honor the memories of those who have already gone before us, taken by this.

God Bless you and I love you all.

I wanted to share my story with all cancer survivors, those who are still fighting pancreatic cancer and anyone who is still "Fighting the Good Fight." Cancer is such a devastating diagnosis, one that changes your life forever. Everyone around you in your life is affected, from your spouse, your family and close friends, and even your co-workers.

I remember the day I got my diagnosis of Stage IIb Neuroendocrine Pancreatic Cancer. Neuroendocrine Pancreatic Cancer is the same cancer that Steve Jobs passed away from. Many people have this and have survived it if caught early. I am a **MEN1** (Multiple Endocrine Neoplasia) gene carrier, which meant that I am prone to endocrine tumors forming in my body. I have already had two parathyroidectomy surgeries, both of them being benign. **MEN1** tumors usually form in the pancreas, parathyroids, and the pituitary.

My pituitary has checked out normal, for which I am very grateful to God! I wanted to share how my Faith has held me during my Fight with pancreatic cancer. If I had waited a few months longer before diagnosis, I would have had to go into palliative care. You will see in my story, how God has been good to me, as He promises!

I dedicate this story to ALL cancer survivors, not just pancreatic cancer patients. We all suffer the same feelings, the same moments of hopelessness and fear when getting the diagnosis. We all wonder at our future, what becomes of us, our bodies, our families, and close friends. There is much to think about when getting a diagnosis.

I wanted to share that since I started this book, I have just recently been diagnosed as "Cancer Free!" God has been good to me…again! I had two malignancies still in my pancreas and 5 years after the Whipple surgery, the last three CT Scans have shown "no evidence of cancer" anywhere, even in the pancreas! We have been dumbfounded, having not done chemotherapy, radiation, or any type of treatment.

Why did they suddenly "disappear?"

Because of my Faith! Because God listened to our prayers.

Welcome to my story and I hope you or your loved one who is fighting pancreatic cancer or any type of cancer, will receive comfort from it.

May God Bless you in your Journey!

Table of Contents

"God will meet you where you are in order to take you where He wants you to go."

- Tony Evans

CHAPTER ONE

Discovery

"Mrs. Burton, your endoscopy shows that you have malignant pancreatic cancer".

I remember those words well. The Gastroenterologist had done an endoscopy to check on the stage and grade of the mass on the head of the pancreas. During the endoscopy procedure, he discovered two other smaller tumors that had spread from the main tumor to the rest of the pancreas and were undetectable during the original CT Scan. The biopsies were sent to the lab for pathology and they were found to be malignant.

But first things first. I'm getting ahead of myself. Let's start with how it got discovered. I thought to myself, "This is a huge test of your Faith. Get ready."

Discovery of the Pancreatic Mass

I had decided to get gastric bypass surgery to lose weight. I had become obese over the years and I was a whopping 291 lbs. I had sleep apnea, Type II diabetes, terrible joint pain in both of my hips, and it was difficult to do normal things like walking through the department store or grocery store without stopping to rest.

I was starting a new life with my husband, who had been my high school sweetheart and we had broken up and gone our separate ways after high school. After 30 years, we reconnected and got married in 2008. It was a good time for us, for we had always loved each other all these years, even when married to others. We considered ourselves very lucky to have found our way back to each other and we wanted to make our life together worthwhile!

I had gained weight over the years and it was causing some health problems. Type II diabetes, taking Metformin for it, joint pain in my hips, and sleep apnea. I also developed breathing problems because we lived in a mountainous city in Northwest Arkansas and the slopes around our house made it difficult to take walks, for it caused breathing problems. After researching for 3 years about Gastric Bypass, I decided to take "the plunge" and to go for it!

It was a very exciting decision and my husband was an avid supporter of this decision, although he always whispered to me that he "loved me no matter what size I was!" What a sweet man!

The gastric bypass procedure was a breeze. No complications and recovery was easy. I was a "model patient" as per my surgeon's words at each monthly appointment. Everyone was happy. The surgeon was pleased with my progress, I was pleased with my new "body", my health was getting better and my husband was happy because I was happy! I bought new clothes and shopping was becoming a fun pastime. All was well until one afternoon on the treadmill.

What happened?

Seven months after my weight loss surgery, I suffered a stabbing pain in my lower right groin area while exercising on my treadmill. Mark suggested that we call my surgeon for a CT Scan to check for a possible hernia. Hernias happen often after gastric bypass surgeries during strenuous exercise because of excess skin pulling on muscles in the lower abdomen. I didn't think much of this and we went to my weight loss surgeon to have the CT Scan and to discuss its findings.

We went out to dinner and waited for the telephone call from my surgeon about the CT Scan results. We live an hour and a half's drive away and he wanted us in the city in case we needed to go into the hospital that night. We went to Olive Garden and were enjoying a nice Italian dinner when Mark's cell rang. He answered it and I watched his face anxiously, wondering what the results were. His face was unreadable until he nodded and thanked the doctor for his call, telling him we would call him first thing in the morning.

He turned to me, took my hands into his and said, "Want the bad news first or the good news first?" Eyes wide, I said, "Of course, I want the good news but what does this mean 'bad news'? I was starting to get nervous, having lost my appetite. "What did he say? Do I have a hernia or not?"

"He said that the CT Scan showed no hernia, but they found a large mass on your pancreas and that it didn't look good. We are to call him in the morning for a referral to a surgeon who specializes in pancreatic surgery." Mark was looking steadily at me as he repeated Dr K.'s words to me, not sure himself what all this meant. The "C" word was never mentioned in this discussion as we were not expecting the word "cancer" to come into the equation at this time.

We finished our dinner and went home in silence, holding hands in the car on the way home, darkness descending upon us as we ascended into the mountains from the city, each of us with our own thoughts.

*"What am I going to do now?
What has happened to me?"*

"God never said that the Journey would be easy, but He did say that the arrival would be worthwhile."

- Max Lucado

CHAPTER TWO

Diagnosis

"Mrs. Burton, your endoscopy shows that you have malignant pancreatic cancer."

When those words were uttered to me by the Gastroenterologist who did the endoscopy and needle biopsy, my heart jumped into my throat. My husband immediately put his arms around me and we both cried. It seemed like the world came to an end; our dreams, our lives we had planned to live together, all came crashing down.

Did you feel that way when you or your loved one received their news? How did you feel? Probably like I did! It's like a feeling of a sinking ship, the Titanic perhaps, her stern going down into the cold, dark ocean after hitting the iceberg that "all of a sudden" appeared out of nowhere. You think to yourself, "Now what? What am I going to do? Shall I do treatment or just let it happen?"

Not just any cancer but *the most lethal kind*: pancreatic cancer. The statistics of surviving pancreatic cancer within 5 years of diagnosis is very low. The most famous case is Patrick Swayze, who battled it like a hero until he succumbed within 2 years after his Stage IV diagnosis. The average survival rate for a Stage III or Stage IV pancreatic cancer is usually within 2 months to a year after diagnosis, depending on treatment options and other variables.

Was that in store for me? Palliative care in a hospice setting, veins pumped with morphine?

Let's move on to something more positive!

In my case, the pancreatic tumor was a 2cm x 3cm mass on the head of my pancreas, in the neuroendocrine islet cells. It was considered a "non-functioning" tumor which meant I had it for several years without symptoms. It was discovered that it had spread to two smaller locations, one in the body and the other in the tail of the pancreas. Stage IIb and low grade aggressiveness with differentiation in the pathology. In a nutshell, all in all, I had malignant tumors in my body that were borderline inoperable and I had to make a decision to either have the tentative option of the Whipple Procedure to remove the head tumor, leaving the other two alone for "monitoring", or just not to do anything at all.

What were my options? Just those two. Chemotherapy and radiation were out of the question for my particular type of cancer. We decided to do the Whipple and have the surgeon "look" at the other two smaller ones to see if they could be "scooped out." It was better than the other option: to leave it alone and let it spread further out into my body so that I would die from it.

What would you do?

I decided to get into the lifeboat and see if I would be rescued. That way, I had a chance at living my life, however it might be. Although my husband and I were practicing Christians, this part of my Christian journey started. My Faith in God really got personal at this juncture and I had to dig deep inside to pull out the strength for fighting this fight.

The Referral

Dr. K___ referred me to a Pancreatic Specialist/Surgeon at a major university teaching hospital in the Midwest. The appointment was made for the following week, which I thought was rather fast considering how hard it was to get in to see this particular surgeon. It was a six-hour drive from Northwest Arkansas to St Louis and we had to stay several days.

Dr. L___ was a very nice man, his demeanor very professional, yet he immediately made me feel comfortable. I was nervous, not knowing what was going on. I had been warned not to get onto the Internet and Google for information, but it's human nature to do just the opposite! I wanted to educate myself on what limited knowledge I had at this point.

During the consultation, I was informed that the CT Scan had shown a "large solid mass of well differentiation on the head of the pancreas" and further testing was needed to confirm whether it was a benign mass or a malignancy. It was agreed that we would do an MRI to see deeper into the mass and to determine if an endoscopy would be needed.

MEN1 Diagnosis

Dr L.___ explained to me that it was definitely a "neoplasm" and asked me about my history of tumors. I explained that I had once been told that I was of the MEN1[1] gene, which is rare but is oftentimes the cause of parathyroid, pituitary, and pancreatic tumors. **Multiple endocrine neoplasia type 1 (MEN1)** is a hereditary condition associated with tumors of the endocrine (hormone producing) glands. **MEN1** was originally known as Werner Syndrome.

The most common tumors seen in **MEN1** involve the parathyroid gland, islet cells of the pancreas, and pituitary gland. Other endocrine tumors seen in MEN1 include adrenal cortical tumors, carcinoid tumors and rarely, pheochromocytomas, as well as tumors in other parts of the digestive tract.

I have already had two prior surgeries to remove three parathyroid tumors from my thyroid (both of which were benign)and, so far, no pituitary tumors had been detected. I also developed a benign tumor in what was left of my thyroid gland and I had surgery to remove the entire thyroid gland (a total thyroidectomy). I also have two small benign adrenal tumors but they do not cause any effects in my body. We just leave them alone. There has been no growth in them for years. I have my prolactin levels checked by blood tests every so often to make certain my pituitary gland is functioning properly.

My father was often hospitalized for large kidney stones and his brother had a total pancreatectomy (complete removal of the pancreas) years ago in the late 1960's. My uncle eventually passed away from complications of the pancreatic removal. The MEN1 gene mutation is usually inherited and given to children through a parent, so it is highly likely that I inherited the **MEN1** gene from my father.

Thanks, Dad! Of course, I didn't blame my father. He had no idea, having passed away 25 years ago. He suffered so much with those kidney stones, it was not a pleasant thing for him. We were a very close family, my mother, father, and myself. Just we three!

Dr L.___ was extremely interested in the **MEN1** diagnosis and explained to me that it could quite possibly be a cancerous tumor but no one would know anything until the MRI and Endoscopy FNA (Fine Needle Aspiration) biopsy could be done. After an initial review of the MRI, an endoscopy FNA was scheduled for the next morning.

I spent that night in prayer, wondering what was in store for me. What if I had pancreatic cancer? Would I live? If I survived, how many years would I live? Would my quality of life be good? Pancreatic cancer is so lethal, having a very low survival rate.

What would you do?

How would you feel if you had to face something like this? A doctor tells you you have cancer. Something so large, an unknown, unexplored area and so scary. I knew that many people have gone through this for different types of cancer and have come through stronger than before. I was hoping that I would be one of those people.

My mother and I often discussed "what we would do" if one of us got cancer, having gone through the loss of her two sisters both to breast cancer and lung cancer. Both died within six months of diagnosis. I often told Mom that if I ever got cancer, I would refuse treatment because of what I observed with their chemotherapy and radiation.

Boy, was I ever wrong. Spoken out of ignorance and perhaps a sense of hopeful bravado that I would never get cancer?

Many questions went through my mind that night in our hotel room bed and I hardly slept. You just never know what is ahead when you are beginning to face something like this. My mother was gone, having passed away suddenly a year before this, and I have no brothers or sisters to lean on.

My husband Mark was the only person in my life that I could depend on, lean on for comfort. Thank God I had him, my best friend, there for support. I also feel that God blessed my mother by bringing her Home before this diagnosis, for she would not have handled it well.

She had been living with heart problems and suffered an aneurysm, surviving that one before she finally suffered a final myocardial heart attack and was gone before she fell to the floor a year before my diagnosis. It would not have been good.

I never felt so frightened in my life until that night.

I could have Pancreatic Cancer.

"If you can't fly, then run. If you can't run, then walk. If you can't walk, then crawl, but whatever you do, you have to keep moving forward."

- Martin Luther King, Jr.

CHAPTER THREE

Treatment and Aftercare

"Not Whipped by The Whipple"

I had my Whipple Surgery two weeks after my diagnosis. Those two weeks were a blur in my mind. I functioned on half of a brain, walking around my home in a daze. My emotions were all over the place. I even started talking about burial plans with my husband in spite of his pleas, of "Please don't talk like that!" You're going to be just fine! You'll see!"

"I'm going to be just fine?" It was nice that someone had a positive outlook at that time because I sure didn't. I was scared, wondering what it would be like to see my wonderful Mother and Father in Heaven, how soon would it be, etc. Would they meet me at the moment my Soul ascends? I don't like to say the word "die."

Your mind takes off on a path of its own, it seems. It races this way and that way, down paths you never thought you would ever think about. My Whipple surgery went without a hitch. The only glitch was that the surgeon, once he reached into my abdomen and did his exploration, saw that it was more advanced than originally thought.

My two smaller tumors were inoperable and could not be taken out. His only options at that moment were to either take the entire pancreas out and reduce my quality of life considerably or remove the larger primary tumor and leave the other two in their places, for monitoring.

This would give me time to live and a chance to have a quality of life and I wouldn't have to do chemotherapy or radiation.

When I was in my room the day after the surgery, he was visiting with me about my options and what the surgery entailed. I asked him the question that we ALL ask: *How long do I have*? I will never forget his demeanor. He was very jovial and he shrugged his shoulders and said, "You're going to be just fine!" You have about a good 10 to 15 years of good quality life!"

10 to 15 years of good quality life? Wow! That was good news to me! Then it dawned on me that I could possibly die after 15 years. I was only 54! That meant I would still be a relatively young woman, not even reaching the age of 70 years. Thinking about this, suddenly solemn, I asked him "Then what?" He replied that there would definitely come a time where I would have to make a decision to have a total removal of my pancreas, thus reducing my quality of life or just leaving it in and go into palliative care to be cared for as it spread.

He explained that with a total removal, my life would reduce to a life of being a Type 1 Diabetic with dependence on insulin shots and wearing a pain pump for pain. Eating would be a chore plus a, "whole host of problems you don't want to think about at this time" to quote him.

Wow. What a future!

I decided that I would take the 10 to 15 years of quality life. I went home after 8 days in the hospital, where I had excellent care and a wondrous crew of nurses and health aides. I didn't have to do chemotherapy or radiation. All I had to do was just start living. God was good to me. Times like this makes your Faith grow stronger.

I would take that! Would you? Of course you would!

The Whipple would not whip me!

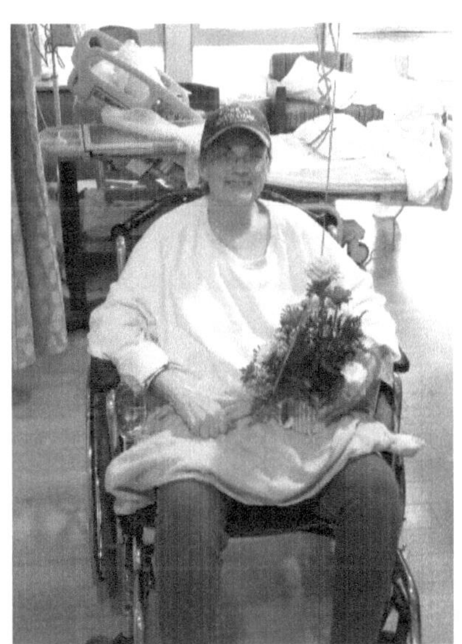

Sarah leaving the hospital

At Home Now

After this intense surgery, we drove the 6 long hours home from the hospital. Once home, I had to think about how I was going to recover at home. What was the next step? My life was turned completely upside-down, not to mention my husband's! He became my sole caregiver 24/7. That is a huge responsibility for a man in all aspects from spiritually to physically. We were fortunate that we were retired at home and didn't have to worry about taking time out from work.

If you work and this happened to you, what would you do?

I often wondered this about other cancer patients, especially those who had inoperable cancer. Do you take out long term disability or completely quit work and go on indefinite disability?

There are many things to consider once diagnosed with malignant cancer.

My husband fixed our bed so that I would be comfortable all day and night. The Whipple is one of the most debilitating surgical procedures to go through and my recovery was extremely painful and difficult. I went against the advice of my surgeon and the anesthesiologist's recommendation to have the epidural and, boy, was it HARD!

Every movement we take so much for granted, such as sitting up or going for a simple walk, became monumental tasks with huge amounts of pain. I had such wonderful care by the very experienced nurses and their aides that I never forgot them and I have wonderful memories of these hard-working people who actually cared about me as a patient. Leaving the hospital with round-the-clock care and coming home to a care giving situation was a big change. I'm sure you or your loved one had to have a relative or friend who became a caregiver. That is a tremendous responsibility for them to take on. It's not just about the patient, it's also about those who become the caregiver.

Let me tell you about the care giving role my husband Mark had to take on.

My Husband The Caregiver

"We gain strength and courage, and confidence by each experience in which we really stop to look fear in the face…we must do that which we think we cannot."
- Eleanor Roosevelt

Mark became my most loving, devoted, and compassionate husband and when the time called for it, he became my sole caregiver. He slid smoothly into the role of care giving, having a "caretaker's" personality. He cooked all our meals, set his alarm for every 2 hours to turn me over in bed, for I couldn't do it without his assistance. He helped me with my medication, fed me my meals that were specially prepared since my pancreas did not digest in the normal way again.

Later in this book, I will talk about how I learned to eat my meals in such a way that I no longer have pain with my remaining pancreas. I will talk about digestive enzymes and how to take them with your meals for the best absorption values.

He assisted me with my personal hygiene in every sense of the word. He gave up his own "life" in a sense of the word to devote all his time to my care and recovery. He suffered bouts of physical fatigue, anger at other people who wouldn't step up to "babysit" me for a couple of hours while he went to the grocery store or any other errands that needed to be done. No one even offered to run an errand or two for him. He suffered a myriad of emotions during that time but kept them to himself as he had a wife who needed him desperately.

The poor man did everything: housework, laundry, cooked the meals, took care of our pets, plus took care of his own needs such as keeping up our two cars, keeping the yard manicured, our flowers watered, all of this on top of taking care of my own recovery needs.

*He did **everything** for that entire year.*

Talk about bonding. This is one of the most bonding times a couple can have and I must say it strengthened our love for each other and deepened it. I started to see how God plays in our lives and that is when I started to see how having malignant pancreatic cancer could have good benefits in my life.

I began to see that having pancreatic cancer deepened my trust in my husband, seeing him with different eyes. I often tell myself that God brought him to me for this purpose, to take care of me during this time. "For Better or Worse," right? Just as I may be called upon to take care of him someday.

Even now, he still has to slip into his care giving mode every so often as I still have days when my cancer gives me pain and I have to take to my bed for a few hours or sometimes a day or two.

It never ends.

This is when the fun starts. Or does this become an "up and down" roller coaster ride? When it becomes that roller coaster ride, how do you get yourself out of it?

Keep reading and I will tell you how *I* did it! God is always Faithful and is always there by your side!

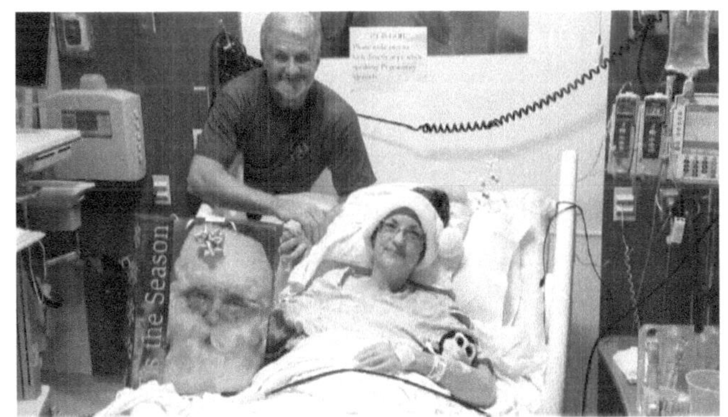

Sarah and her husband Mark in her hospital room.
Christmas 2014

A Myriad of Emotions: The Beginning of the Roller Coaster Ride

Once the shock wore off from the actual diagnosis of my inoperable malignancy and I had time to lie in bed thinking about things, the roller coaster ride of emotions began for me. They say that when we lose a loved one, we go through stages of grief. I can say that it was the same for me. It is like grief in its own way, grief in the thought that I could die soon and leave my husband behind. Grief at the loss of dreams and plans that we had made together, dreams and plans such as traveling in an RV across the United States and a European trip or two.

Grief at the loss of a person: the person I was before the diagnosis.

It's like experiencing similar feelings upon the death of a loved one. You lose that part of yourself that you knew, the part of yourself that knew when you got up each morning, you could achieve certain plans that you made that day without worrying about a health problem. The part of yourself that you now realize is no longer there or "no longer alive" in a sense of the word. It's a terrible emotion to have. The realization that the departed loved one is a *part of you.*

Learning to Live and Feel Alive

*"The best and most beautiful things in this world
cannot be seen or even heard, but must be felt
with the heart."*
- Helen Keller

What a beautiful statement. Helen Keller was deaf and blind so, naturally, she could not see nor hear. The only thing she could do was feel. As a deaf woman, I can relate to this because we tend to feel emotions on a deeper level. We feel emotions deeply because we cannot hear. Our expressions come from the written word or with a flick of the hand during an ASL (American Sign Language) "conversation." I am currently learning how to do ASL with my husband but I can speak normally and express in voice how I think and feel. I thought it appropriate to insert this at this point for this is all about feeling what we feel when we are diagnosed.

Anyway, back to the discussion at hand!

You start to get into the "introspective" side of yourself. Maybe you were not a introspective sort of person before your diagnosis. Maybe you were a very poetic person.

It can be easy to overcompensate at this point. Grief comes in many forms. I am a deaf woman and artist with a studio in my home. I have dreams of going to art shows with my husband, working on painting furniture and other types of artwork. Getting up each morning, taking my coffee to my studio and getting right to work, very mundane activities we all do every day.

As the months went by, I spent so many days in bed. All day long, with Mark being my caregiver, plus we had a Home Health Care Nurse who came by three times per week to check vitals and status of pain management control. This gave me a lot of time to lie and think about things, ponder my life as it currently was and how was I going to get through it.

Mark started buying me books by **Joel Osteen** and **Joyce Meyer**, inspirational books about getting through a tough situation. I read those books through and through, going back and forth within their paragraphs as I tried to understand their message. I often wondered why God allowed this to happen to me. What was the purpose? What did He want me to learn? I am sure I will find out!

When you are faced with a life or death situation such as this, you start to ponder about why this happened to you. I asked God, "Why me?" I asked Him why this happened to me, why did I have to have cancer, not only cancer per se but *inoperable* cancer! However, that is partly true. In order to be completely cancer free, I would have to have a pancreatectomy (total removal of the pancreas).

If I did that, my life would certainly be different. The quality of life would not be as good as it is now after I recovered from my surgery. I am not sure I want to do that, to be honest. My uncle lived without a pancreas for a short time, about 3 to 5 years from what I remember as a small child. Not much was spoken about his illness, for it was not known back then as it is now.

"Why Me, God?"

I certainly asked that question every day. Each day when I couldn't get out of bed, befuddled by strong pain medication. The Whipple is a hard operation to recover from, more so because I didn't have the epidural. If I had had the epidural, I would have been able to sit up in bed and walk more often than I did, and earlier in the recovery process after the surgery.

The pain was tremendous and the emotions flickering through my mind, questioning my spirituality, questioning God, doing the "Why me?" thing. I was wondering if this was something that I was supposed to learn something from. What was I supposed to learn? Humility? Compassion? Empathy for others who are going/or have gone through the same thing?

It came to me that I was supposed to learn more about my relationship with God. I was always a Christian but I went to church sporadically because of my deafness. It was difficult to sit in a pew and read the minister's lips from a distance. Now, I am going through a very difficult situation in my life and I could have died.

I didn't, though. They say that, "God wasn't finished with me." Maybe I was supposed to learn about my *own* personal relationship with God and where it was at this time of my life.

My relationship with God became stronger and more personal on a deeper level

"There is no one who is insignificant in the purpose of God"

-Alistair Begg

CHAPTER FOUR

Now What?

Survivor's Guilt

What do I do with myself as I lie in bed all day, 23 hours out of the 24 hour day. The only time I got up was to go to the restroom, shower with help from Mark and a few times when I would go out into the living room to watch TV with my husband. Mark did everything he could to help me walk and covered me up with blankets in the recliner, Frida lying on my lap. Frida is our Chihuahua and she loves to lay on Mama's lap. Frida got lots of loving at that time!

As I lay in bed, I was able to look out our bedroom window which had a wonderful view of the mountains in front of our house. Our house sat on the side of a mountain in Northwest Arkansas and had a gorgeous view. I would often lie on my side and look out that window, pondering about things. I had so much time to think!

My husband would get the newspaper and bring it to me to read. Every once in awhile, an obituary would be printed about someone who passed away from pancreatic cancer.

I found myself bursting into tears every time I would read an obituary of someone who passed from pancreatic cancer. I found myself asking God, "Why am I still alive and that person isn't?" Oftentimes when someone is diagnosed with pancreatic cancer, it is usually caught at a late stage and they would pass away within a few months. That was hard to read about. I cried for those people.

They say this is "Survivor's Guilt." People who are sole survivors of plane crashes or car crashes often talk about the guilt they feel that they are still alive and the others involved in that crash were killed. That is how I felt whenever I would read about someone passing away from pancreatic cancer, especially one who only lived a very short time after diagnosis.

I learned that Survivor's Guilt can be a good thing because it makes us more in touch with our own mortality. Perhaps it would make us more humble. It would make us more compassionate towards others. It would make us have more empathy for others who suffer an illness or a hard time in their life.

Life as an Only Child

I was an only child, raised by very loving parents who had me late in life, and they doted on me. My mother felt guilt because I was born deaf. There was no physical reason that I was born deaf. No one in my family was deaf. I found myself thinking about my deafness, the bullying I went through in school, and how people treated me throughout my life. I learned to talk through speech therapy and went to public school from kindergarten to graduation, going on to college later in life to pursue an arts degree.

Life was different in the late 1950's and 1960's for the deaf culture. We didn't have the awareness in society then as we do today. My parents were unable to put me into a deaf school because this would have involved a large move to another city several hours away from family and a changing of jobs for my father.

The decision was made for me to go to public school and I was the only "handicapped" child among "normal" children. Life was very difficult for me. My parents tried very hard to shelter me from painful experiences and I often ran home crying, running into my bedroom and shutting the door to shut everyone out. I turned to art and music, which became my best friends. I was able to hear music via hearing aids.

Living with deafness in the "hearing world" was a battle because I had to learn everything from a hearing person's point of view. Nothing was ever spoken or "learned" about things from a deaf person's point of view.

Nothing was ever spoken or "learned" about things from a deaf person's point of view. Sitting on the front row at school so that I could lip read the teacher sometimes would make someone accuse me of being the teacher's pet.

That was so far from the truth! Somehow I made it through elementary school in the 1960's and the early 1970's saw me go into junior high grades 7th through 9th. This was in the early 1970's when marijuana was beginning to be rampant in the schools and everyone wanted to be like Janis Joplin or Rod Stewart or whoever their favorite rock musician was.

I was not part of that crowd, so I suffered severe bullying from classmates. My parents took me out of that school and we moved to the country where we could have some privacy.

I ended up in a small town school and it was better. I was able to have a horse and I discovered a latent ability to "communicate" with horses and just fell in love with them! I ended up learning how to train Quarter Horses for showing and barrel racing.

I won trophies and had lots of ribbons. This went a long way to restoring self confidence in myself as a person with my own identity. I was very athletic as I helped my father with hefting those heavy hay bales into the iron feeders every day, building up those muscles in my arms!

In High School, I met my current husband and he was such a cutie then! This was when the guys all had long hair and mine was long and black, much like Cher's. They used to call me "Pocahontas" because I tanned so dark during the summer riding horses. Oh, those were the days! Those were good years for me as I was so healthy and athletic. Having pancreatic cancer was something never imagined in those days.

After I graduated High School in 1977, I went on to live a life of normalcy, getting married, working as a Graphic Designer for the Avionics Industry such as Boeing and Cessna Aircraft Companies.

I lived in Los Angeles and Seattle for a while before coming back home to Kansas. In the Fall 2000 Semester, I enrolled at Wichita State University to start a path to obtaining a Bachelor's of Fine Arts degree in Studio Painting but I dropped out due to the first of my many surgeries: a benign growth on my parathyroid.

That was the beginning of the MEN1 diagnosis.

I think having pancreatic cancer has made me a better person today. I had to grow up!!

How Pancreatic Cancer has made me "Grow Up"

*"I got the guts to die…but I wanna know if you got
the guts to live!"*
- Big Daddy, *Cat on a Hot Tin Roof*

Living with pancreatic cancer has opened my eyes to a whole other universe, so to speak. Pancreatic cancer made me realize that life can be short, that I could not live as long as someone of my age with good health. I have realized that I am more empathetic, have more compassion, and definitely have more patience!

I have more responsibility now. I have dreams that I want to achieve and living with cancer has made me more in touch with myself. I have more desire to live and experience more things. I find myself wanting to branch out more in the art field, such as experimenting with different kinds of paint products and painting styles. It has made me more appreciative of my husband, how he feels each day, and just being there with him.

Experiencing his pain when he has pain and emotions, sharing his thoughts and feelings with him. I appreciate his love that much more than the day I married him, if that is possible! Living with malignant cancer has strengthened our love for each other. We appreciate being together and our arguments are minor, more like *discussions* that get resolved quickly.

It is possible to grow from living with malignant cancer. I know, because I am living it. I appreciate life more. I appreciate waking up each day, rising out of bed to start my day in a normal way. I lived an entire year in bed and now I don't want to waste time doing that anymore.

I want to live! You would, too!

"Nevertheless, with God, All Things are Possible!"

- Matthew 19:26

CHAPTER FIVE

Today is the Day is the First Day of the Rest of Your Life!

"*A Reminder: You are not just a Survivor, You are a <u>Thrive-er</u>!*"
- Mark Burton

Soon after recovering, I often found myself making promises to God. Promises such as I would live a better, healthier life. I would be more compassionate of others. I would be a better wife to my husband. I would be a more patient person. A thousand promises.

But you don't have to "make promises" to God to have a good recovery. He is already there beside you, each day, when you get out of bed to walk a little bit. A few steps each day to gain your strength back. He is there beside you each step of the way.

He is there when you cry with pain or frustration. Frustration that perhaps you didn't walk as far as you thought you could. Frustration at anything you set for yourself while lying in bed recovering.

Well, I have good news! You don't have to be frustrated! Recovery is just that…recovering in bed for a few months while your body heals from the very serious surgical procedure to remove all or part of your cancer. While you are recovering, you can be reading inspirational books like I did. I read books ranging from inspirational to crime/forensic thrillers.

I got very frustrated because I would see my husband outside working in our gorgeous front yard, the birds singing as they fluttered around our feeders. I wanted to go outside so bad it was painful!

Then I thought to myself: "If I am wanting to go outside so bad, maybe I am recovering enough that I can go outside!" I would haul myself out of bed with Mark's help and he would assist me out to our front porch to sit in our comfortable rocking porch chairs.

I turned my face towards the sun, feeling the warmth on my face. The warmth of Nature and of God. God had kept me alive in spite of the odds against me. It was a huge step towards my recovery! Not just physically, but to my mind and my Spirit. It was a beautiful moment!

That is when I knew that I was ready to get better and to start thinking of how to fulfill my "new" Life. I started thinking of ways to live as though I did not have malignancies in my body. Ways to live in my *"new normal"* in such a happy and healthy life!

This is when Survivors call their New Birthday, which means Feb 14th, 2014, was my new Birthday. That was the day I became not just a Survivor but a ***Thrive-er***! I sometimes still cry to this day as I remember this:

I am a Survivor and a Thrive-er. Now it's time to make my dreams come true! God wants to restore you. He wants you to have everything He wants for you.

Time to thrive!

A Lesson from Frida Kahlo

"I never painted my dreams. I only painted my own reality."
- Frida Kahlo (1907 - 1954)

As an artist, I was always fascinated by **Frida Kahlo**, a Mexican artist who painted during the Era of Surrealism, an art movement that was popular in the early 1920's and was known for its abstract visual artworks and writings. Frida Kahlo came into prominence in this time with her bold, vibrant colors and her tumultuous relationship with Diego Rivera, a prominent Mexican Fresco painter. I named my Chihuahua, Frida, after her.

As a child, Frida had polio and she suffered a bus accident which left her with multiple serious injuries to her upper torso and pelvic area. She began her painting during this time, wearing a body cast, trying to help herself in her recovery. She was not about to let herself lie in bed and fade away. As they often say, "Mind over Matter."

Her paintings became her method of recovery and this is where I draw my inspiration from her. Not so much her style of painting but the manner in which she painted *through* her pain. I can only imagine what it was like for her.

Can you imagine the suffering of pain she went through while trying to apply her brush to the canvas, struggling to sit up in that body cast?

It is said that she also painted lying on her back, still in the cast, with the canvas above her in a specially constructed cover over her bed.

When I watched the movie "**Frida**" with actress **Salma Hayek** playing the title role, I was transfixed by how she portrayed Frida painting during her pain, her body tight in a body cast. She bit through her pain, pulling each brush stroke of paint across that canvas, grimacing with each stroke. Yet, she persevered. I was enthralled by that, being a painter myself.

That is true dedication! That is sheer willpower of a woman who suffered debilitating pain for years and yet turned out paintings that are now worth millions of dollars. The lesson here is that *she wanted to live each day*, painting, no matter how bad her pain.

With medications available to us as cancer patients today, we can each do something that we love whether it's painting, sewing, knitting/crochet, or any other type of activity that we loved to do before our diagnosis.

Even write a book!

As a cancer survivor still living with malignancies, I often have days that I can't paint but on the days I do paint, I really appreciate it. Sometimes it takes quite a bit of effort on a mental level but I can't let it stop me. Art and writing are my life and I can't live without them. I don't want to!

If Frida Kahlo could paint wearing a body cast, her mind befuddled with strong doses of morphine, then I am sure I can use art as my inspiration for recovery of my mind, body, and soul!

This is a woman that I can admire for her tenacity and her strong sense of story-telling through her paintings which have bold and vibrant colors. It tells me that I could strengthen myself in my recovery by trying to see the world as she saw it.

Creative Visualization can apply to YOU in your recovery. Look up books on this subject and you will find applications on mind and body with which you can function through your malignancy and live a very positive, happy life. Look at what activities you loved to do before your diagnosis and see if that is something you can *still* do in spite of your diagnosis. What a way to improve your mind, body and soul!

I love Art and I decided I was going to use it to help me in my recovery!

How I Found Fulfillment in my Days

After learning lessons from Frida Kahlo's life with pain, I asked myself "What makes me happy?" Of course, I love my husband and pleasing him makes me happy. Making sure he is happy makes me happy. But what of MYSELF? When you have your first "Birthday," (the first year after your diagnosis) you begin to think about yourself and what you can do to make yourself happy.

You may find that things that you thought made you happy before your diagnosis are no longer important in the grand scheme of things. Maybe you weren't a spiritual person before. You may find yourself becoming more spiritual, however you find it. It doesn't matter to God how you find it. As long as you find it, for when you find it, you find Him.

Living with malignancies as I do makes me take stock of what is important in my own life. I discovered that *living as healthy as I can was important.* Dietary changes (both big and small), daily lifestyle changes, and mental changes were very important. Being with my husband as often as I could became important. My artwork and broadening its horizons became very important to me.

Making my studio a happy place of music and creativity became important to me. Loving my little pets became important to me. Right now, my little Parrotlet named Twizzell is sitting in his cage that is pulled up next to my desk as I write this book.

Music plays from the computer speakers and he just sings his little heart out as I reach out my finger, poking it between the bars of the cage and he snakes down towards my finger, ducking his head as if to say "Gimme Scritches, Mommie!" That is now very important to me! Time spent with my family. My relationships with my husband and my pets, although very good before diagnosis, became much more meaningful afterwards.

There are days that I "forget" I have malignant pancreatic cancer. It's a wonderful feeling to have at times!

How Living with My Malignancies Strengthened our Marriage

"Just for Today, Be Happy. Know that you are Loved, just the way you are! As you forgive me, I forgive you. God does not make junk!"
- Mark Burton

Another thing that became very apparent in my life with malignancies was my time on Earth. How much time did I have before God calls me Home? No one knows the answer to that question, so what do you do? You make the best of what time you have left! One thing that has happened is this: my husband got the fright of his life, the sudden, cold knowledge that I could leave him behind, to live alone. Alone without his wife, the wife he had so many good times with, the girl with the long black hair that he loved to look at across the row in Study Hall in high school. A thousand memories that have been made throughout our time together, he could be left alone with. Not a pleasant thought, is it?

I know that many people have gone through that and there are many who have been "left behind" by their spouse. It's a sobering thought. It's a painful thought. I saw it happen to my mother when my father suddenly died of a heart attack.

It was a very painful process for my mother and me; the grief was intense. My mother and father had the kind of marriage in which they always did things together and always told each other that they would "go together."

It was sad to see my Mother suffer in her grief. She never truly recovered, although she lived her remaining 17 years as best as she could, continuing her activities.

That is why I wanted to be a better wife to my husband while I am here. Although I thought I was a good wife before the diagnosis, there is always room for improvement! Our marriage now is wonderful and good. Very happy and fulfilling.

I know that when the day comes that I go Home, I know in my heart that I was loved. Now, let's talk about how we can improve our daily lives with dietary changes in our pancreatic cancer journey.

"When you change your diet, you change your entire physiology and you can heal!"

- Charlotte Gerson, *"As The Healing Effect"*

CHAPTER SIX

Helpful Diet Plans for Pancreatic Cancer

How a Proper Diet Improved My Life

My meals were changed drastically by the Whipple surgery, in a large way. It was a very hard journey for me to get to where I am now. I can eat "comfortably" now without pain but I have learned how to stay away from certain foods. If I ate those certain foods, I was in for a "rough ride" and usually a trip to the ER for pain relief and CT Scans. I would take to my bed with painkillers for 3-5 days to recover. It was rough!

So, I decided to really take a long, hard look at my dietary needs and see which foods were the "bad guys" and the ones that were "the good guys."

Foods that contain high amounts of fat were the culprits that led to those ER trips. If you have had the Whipple, your pancreas can no longer digest high amounts of fat as it did before. I discovered that not only could it not digest high amounts of fat, it also couldn't handle high glucose foods. The "sugar dumping" was horrendous; it put me to bed for several hours with nausea and palpitations. "Fat Dumping" does the same thing, so be very careful!

It is very important to recognize your body's reactions to certain foods.

It's imperative to your healing process that you understand this.

When I had my gastric bypass surgery, I had to go through 6 months of Nutritional Counseling. I learned about the benefits of high protein and low carb diets and how it works with the "new plumbing" in my body. The Roux-N-Y procedure is very similar to the Whipple and since I had that done before my Whipple, I already had a diet plan in place and my body was already used to the change in dietary foods. My surgeon didn't think I needed digestive enzymes since I was already eating a "whipple diet" with the gastric bypass dietary needs.

As it turned out, this was a mistake! I needed digestive enzymes and my body suffered!

I went a whole year without using digestive enzymes and I must admit that it was not pleasant. Not using enzymes with each meal causes various problems such as improper digestion and severe pain caused by gas build-up in your intestines. Flatulence became a huge problem and it was very embarrassing! It got to where I wouldn't go out of the house and became home-bound. It was not a pleasant lifestyle!

Solaray's Pancreatin 1300 - My Dietary Best Friend!

I went to see an Oncologist to get some answers to my digestion problems and he suggested that I get on Procrease, a pharmaceutical grade digestive enzyme capsule, taking 2 or 3 per meal each day. Or even Creon. However, the one problem I had was my medical insurance would not cover the $450-per-month prescription! Creon was even more expensive: $800 per month co-pay! I had to get onto Google to do a massive search for a digestive enzyme that would work for my budget.

I came up with Pancreatin 1300 manufactured by Solaray Vitamins, one of my favorite vitamin supplements. I find Solaray to be consistent with their supplements, so based on my past history with Solaray vitamins, I got the Pancreatin.

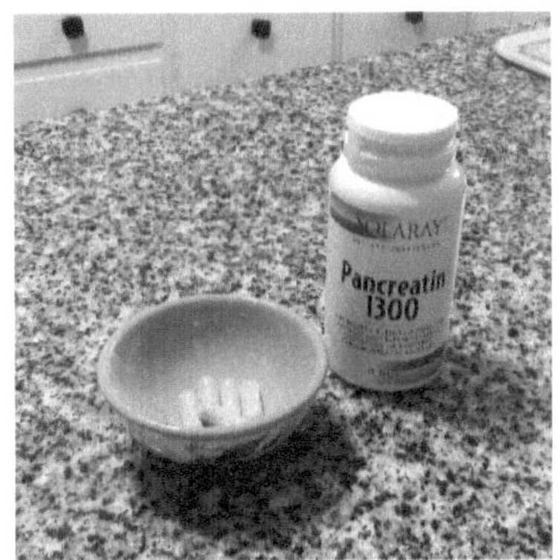

Photo courtesy of Sarah Burton

Each capsule in Pancreatin 1300 has a blend of the important supplements used in digestion: Lipase, Amylase, and Protease. It helps improve digestion of carbohydrates, protein, and fats. What is most important is that Lipase is the ingredient used to break down the fats that the pancreas cannot do after surgery. I take 5 capsules of Pancreatin with each meal and it is wonderful. It really helps and the price is great! I buy it from *Vitacost.com* at $20.11 for 2 bottles. I use 4 bottles per month. The flatulence is non-existent when the supplements are taken properly and there is no more pain caused by "flare-ups" of the pancreas, often diagnosed as *pancreatitis*. No more hospital visits for that!

It sure is nice!

Let's look at some examples of meal planning in which I used my pancreatin and explore the importance of Protein Shakes and Smoothies.

The Importance of Protein Shakes and Smoothies

Also, I must note that I also drink protein shakes made with a mixture of **Unjury Protein Powder** (Chocolate Splendor Flavor or Strawberry flavor) which is medical grade protein powder, a frozen fruit such as strawberries or blueberries, and 8 oz of nonfat Light Greek Yogurt. Here is the recipe:

- Unjury Protein Powder (www.unjury.com - There are many flavors to choose from!)
- 8oz of Nonfat Greek Yogurt Vanilla Flavored (or any flavor you desire)
- 4oz of frozen fruit of your choice
- 4oz of ice
- A dash of Vanilla Extract
- 2 Splenda packets for sweetening.

This makes a wonderful protein shake/smoothie and it's very filling. You don't need to take Pancreatin digestive enzymes with this because it's very, very low in fat. Eat foods low in fats!

Eating Foods Low in Fat

Eating foods low in fats guarantee good digestive health after pancreatic cancer surgery. It is very important to do this. Research your favorite foods and see what their fat contents are. These are my favorites and I was astounded at what I discovered about the fat content of each one. I learned this when I had my Gastric Bypass nutritional counseling which made it very helpful for my dietary needs after the Whipple surgery. I ate the following in small quantities:

- Deli meats such as smoked turkey, oven roasted turkey. Beef is all right but remember, it's higher in fat.
- Soups such as Progresso Home Style Chicken & Noodles (Heart Light)
- Eggs (scrambled or over easy). After surgery, it is a good idea to purée your eggs for a month or so after the Whipple
- Multi Grain bread (one slice). It's good for fiber as you need it for digestive help.
- Go easy on butter and oils. My favorite oil is Olive Oil,(Extra Virgin, cold-pressed). It's so good for your stomach and very healthy.
- Light Mayo is permitted. I had this on one slice of multi-grain bread (one light swipe) with a piece of cheese or a deli meat.

No chips of any kind. It is hard for your "new" stomach to digest and can cause pain. I eat Club Crackers in place of this and it's so tasty! Makes a great snack for between meals to keep your strength and blood sugar up.

Sample Meals that are easy on the Pancreas

Over time, my husband has figured out how to cook for me while I was bed-bound after surgery. I have discovered that this was the best way for me to eat if I wanted to avoid an attack of pancreatitis or even a pain in the pancreas. I have listed some meal samples that I have had success with:

Sample Breakfast Meals:

- 1/2 cup of Old Fashioned Oatmeal cooked 5 mins
- One slice of multi-grain or sourdough bread
- 1 pat of lowfat margarine. I like to use Brummel & Brown; it's butter made with yogurt. Very smooth and low in fat
- 1 cup of decaf coffee, with non dairy creamer and Splenda. Sugar is hard on the newly surgical stomach because if you had a Whipple, you may have had a Roux En Y procedure done, which means your sugar intake needs to change to sugar substitutes to avoid "dumping."
- Scrambled eggs made with lowfat milk
- One slice of toasted multi-grain or sourdough bread
- 1 pat of lowfat margarine

- 3 or 4 slices of turkey bacon or sausage. I use turkey because it's lower in fat than bacon. It's great for protein just like pork bacon and much better for you fat-wise.
- One slice of toast (multi-grain or sourdough bread)
- 1 pat of lowfat margarine
- 1 or 2 eggs, soft boiled (or hardboiled, whichever is your preference).
- Light salting for the eggs.

As time goes on after your surgery, I was able to eat "lightly fluffed" hash browns (light, not crispy) with my toast and turkey bacon or sausage. I always try to keep my portion control to 1 cup total of the dinner selections (1/2 cup of each selection)because it keeps the pancreas from going into "overdrive" in the digestive process and keeps the blood sugar levels controlled.

Sample Lunch Meals:

- One slice of multi-grain or sourdough bread
- One slice of cheese of your choice (I use one slice of Velveeta!)
- One swipe of Light Mayo or condiment of your choice.
- One slice of lettuce. Romaine, iceberg, or any of your choice.
- One 8 ounce diet soda, lowfat milk, or G-2/low sugar Gatorade. I drink G-2 because of my ulcer and it works for me.

- Protein Shake. (See above for Protein shake recipe). Protein shakes may be made with 1/2 cup of frozen fruit of your choice, a banana, or even a teaspoon of peanut butter for flavoring! Check with your local nutrition store or even with Unjury Protein if you buy from them. They have wonderful lists for different flavoring for Protein shakes to make it fun and tasty. Even Holiday Season flavorings! You can buy books that have Smoothie recipes for variety in taste.

- Chef salad (small portion) with Olive Oil. Balsamic vinaigrette was good for awhile until I developed a peptic ulcer, which is common after Whipple surgery or Roux En Y procedures. Mine happened 6 years after my surgery and it was an extremely painful process to heal. You can always add meat of your choice, cheeses, and other vegetables to your salad to make it interesting and tasty. I always like to add black olives and red onion to my salads. Makes it interesting! Sometimes the red onion makes it hard to kiss my husband afterwards!

If romance is in the air, maybe skip the red onion or take a rinse of your mouth with a mouthwash after the salad . . .!

Sample Dinner Meals:

- Healthy Choice, Smart Choice or Lean Cuisine Meal Dinner.
- 1/2 cup of a vegetable of your choice.
- One slice of multi-grain or sourdough bread
- 1 pat of lowfat margarine

- Grilled Seafood (shrimp, lobster, scallops, salmon, etc) or grilled chicken. Very good for you, full of protein, and low in fat. I eat a lot of seafood, especially when we go out to dinner at Red Lobster or a steak place. Red meat is okay, but not highly recommended because of the "marbling" of fat throughout the meat.
- 1/2 cup Rice Pilaf or Wild Rice. White rice is high in the glycemic index and can cause your blood sugar to go up because of the digestive nature of white rice. Dieticians and Nutritionists always talk about rice and its glycemic properties. Wild rice, brown rice, and rice pilaf are much better for your digestion and it's always highly recommended.

- 1/2 cup of pasta. They are always a good idea to cook it "al fresco" (slightly soft) for it makes it easier to digest with your enzymes.

It's a good idea to get gluten-free pasta because of its ease of digestion.

- Marinara or herb sauce. Cream sauces are high in fat and it's heck on your pancreas. It causes "dumping" and it's a very uncomfortable feeling that lasts about 2-3 hours, so I stay away from any sauce that is "thick and white." Herb sauces, garlic sauces are good and delicious in taste.
- One slice of sourdough bread or if you are eating at Olive Garden, it's okay to have a breadstick or two. I have never had trouble with their breadsticks and I always dip in Olive oil. As I mentioned above, stay away from the balsamic and if this sounds unpalatable to you, you can just have the breadstick by itself if eating at Olive Garden, or sourdough bread with lowfat margarine if cooking it at home.

Desserts are usually not an option because of the high sugar content BUT. . . I have "cheated" and taken a few bites of my husband's desserts!

Protein is your Pancreas' Best Friend

These are all sample meals that I eat with no digestion problems. It has been a journey of trial and error, with many times of "dumping" and writhing in bed with pain, doubled over. There have been times when I went to the ER with a bout of pancreatitis brought on by a meal that was too high in fat. You can buy cookbooks with recipes and I often browse through *Cooking Light*, a diabetic foods magazine that has wonderful recipes that are fun and easy to prepare. Not to mention great on your pancreas. Your pancreas will love it!

I also try to make certain that I have a protein shake at night if I have had a light dinner meal. Keeping my protein intake high helps balance the blood sugar and maintains a healthy metabolism, which is so important in your pancreatic (or any kind of cancer) cancer recovery journey.

Protein helps build muscle mass, strengthens your vascular system, and builds up your red blood cells, imperative for your immune system. The protein shake at night can just be a light one, made with the protein powder and lowfat milk, shaken not stirred. It's so good for your body, for its healing during recovery and beyond.

When my husband and I go out to eat, most restaurants are very helpful when ordering. I have never had problems with ordering "specialized" meals, usually asking for grilled chicken or seafood of my choice, salad with olive oil, and a vegetable on the side.

I don't even order straight from the menu; usually I just browse the menu for what they have as dinner choices and then I discuss meal options with the waitperson. I have never had problems with them looking at me as if I were an alien from outer space.

Sometimes I tell them that I am a pancreatic cancer survivor and have digestive issues, which usually satisfies them and my meal gets planned. I remember after being released from the hospital and we started venturing out to dinner at restaurants, being very nervous and anxious about how to eat. Time has taught me that it is not a problem and now I enjoy eating out, for most restaurants serve the usual: chicken or seafood, salad and a vegetable side!

Cancer doesn't have to be your enemy. It's a fact of our lives when we are survivors and our meals are so important in maintaining a healthy lifestyle after your cancer diagnosis. In fact, today, I don't even think about it anymore. God has made certain that cancer is not my enemy and He has my best interests at heart!

God is your Best Friend and He promises to give you "beauty for ashes" for your pain and mourning.(Isaiah 61:3). He gave me mine and I will now talk about that in the next chapter! A Miracle happened...

"To appoint unto them that mourn in Zion, to give unto them beauty for ashes, the oil of joy for mourning, the garment of praise for the spirit of heaviness; that they might be called trees of righteousness, the planting of the LORD, that He might be Glorified."

- Isaiah 61:3 *King James Version*

CHAPTER SEVEN

Beauty for Ashes - Isaiah 61:3

My Miracle Happened through Faith!

My Beauty for Ashes happened! The Miracle that I never thought would ever happen to me. I had read inspirational books, prayed to God for Him to help me get through my dark times during my cancer journey, etc.

"What happened?" you ask?

Well, I will tell you! I had developed a complication from my gastric bypass surgery which resulted in a peptic ulcer. Apparently the gastric bypass and the Whipple were done pretty close to each other time-wise (less than a year apart) and they caused some problems.

I started having pain in my upper abdomen and we all thought it was pancreatitis. I went to the ER numerous times because of this pain and, given my pancreatic cancer history, it was naturally assumed that I had pancreatitis. CT Scans were done those times, showing nothing "out of character" but my red blood count was high, meaning I was inflamed in my abdomen.

I went into the hospital for an EGD Scope and the scope found that I had a peptic ulcer caused by a leakage in my gastric bypass surgical incision in my stomach below the "pouch." I was treated for it and after 7 weeks, it healed up.

But I still had pain in my abdomen and no one could figure out why. I finally went to a renowned pancreatic cancer oncologist/surgeon in my city and he ran a deep scan pancreatic protocol CT Scan. He was confused as the results showed. . .you said it! No cancer. He asked me several times why did I think I had pancreatic cancer at all? I was flabbergasted!

He got records from my surgeon in New York and from Barnes Jewish Hospital in St Louis where my Whipple was performed and those records said I had Stage IIb Neuroendocrine Pancreatic Cancer.

Another CT Scan was done at another time, still no evidence of cancer. I went to the Oncologist that was referred by this surgeon and visited with him.

He said to me: "Sarah, you have no evidence of cancer in your pancreas or anywhere in your body."

WHAT?? WHAT DID HE JUST SAY TO ME??
Oh my Lord! Did he just tell me that I had no cancer in my body?

He said, smiling and very patiently, "Mrs. Burton, that is correct. You have no evidence of cancer."

Does this mean I am "cancer free?"

He smiled warmly and nodded his head, "Yes. You are now cancer free. I don't know how this happened because tumors don't 'disappear', which is apparently what happened here." Tumors do not "just disappear."

Tumors do not just disappear. Then. . .where did they go? What happened to them? As the Oncologist quietly slipped out of the consultation room, my gaze was locked onto the rainy clouds outside the window in his office. A tear started to roll down my cheek as I suddenly realized the implication of his words.

Cancer free. No evidence of pancreatic cancer. Tumors just. . . Disappeared. Yes, they did.

I burst into tears, crying hard and my husband wrapped me in his arms. I walked to the window to look outside some more, and it seemed to me that the clouds pulled apart, exposing bright blue sky. The sun came out!

I smiled and said to God: "I am now cancer free because of You. You healed me. You gave me Beauty for Ashes because of my pain, my mourning, my dark times. Now it's time for me to LIVE"

What happened? Faith happened. That is what happened. Faith, my long dark journey with my pancreatic cancer strengthened my Faith in God. He is All. He is the Author and the Finisher in my life story. I have things to do with my new life now. I have my husband to live the rest of my life with now.

This is my Beauty for Ashes, my new Life restored to me by God, my Testimony through Mercy and Faith. I have a story and testimony to tell.

Yes, it can happen to you. Look to Him and He will carry you during your journey.

God Bless you.

Thank you, God.

The End
(and a new beginning!)

ACKNOWLEDGMENTS

I want to thank the administrative staff, doctors, and nurses at Siteman Cancer Center in St Louis, Missouri and Wilmot Cancer Center in Rochester, NY for their compassion, optimism, and excellent care of me while I was undergoing my pancreatic cancer surgery and treatments.

I want to thank my editor, Elizabeth T. Greer, an author herself, for her mentorship, advice and encouragement to get me started on this journey of writing this book.

I want to thank Karen E., a fellow pancreatic cancer survivor, for giving me the encouragement and courage to write this book. Her enthusiasm in asking "When is this book coming out?" was infectious!

I want to thank all my writing friends, especially Frank G, who have helped me "hone my skills" in our writing group by having fun with our storylines since 1995.

I want to thank Roller Weight Loss in Fayetteville, Arkansas for their diligence and kindness when the cancer mass was first discovered by them and for their swift action in referring and securing me an appointment with my Surgeon.

I want to thank my Pancreatic Cancer Surgeon, Dr. L, at Wilmot Cancer Center in the University of Rochester, Rochester, NY, for his compassion, expertise in his field and wonderful care of me during my surgeries.

I want to thank my best friend and loving husband, Mark, for his persistence in making sure I was taken to all of my hospital visits, doctor/surgeon appointments, both local and out of state, making me a bed in the back of our SUV for my comfort while he drove us on a 3-day drive to Rochester, NY to the Wilmot Cancer Center for surgical care. His 24/7 aftercare of me is unmatched, greatly appreciated and his ability to put aside his own needs to take care of mine first and foremost for the entire year I spent in bed in severe pain. I love you, sweetheart and I am so thankful to God that I have you!

... and above all, I want to thank God for His Mercy and His Love, standing by me and healing me. He taught me about Faith and how Faith is so important during our trying times. I want to thank Him for giving me the desire to help others and the little seed in my heart to write this book. I give Him Praise!

I INVITE YOU TO VISIT THESE PAGES
FOR UPDATES
AND TO COMMENT ON THIS BOOK:

Facebook:
www.facebook.com/authorsarahburton/
Email: booksbysarahburton@gmail.com

I also invite you to visit the Pancreatic Cancer Action Network website at www.pancan.org. It is a wonderful site full of resources and information about Pancreatic Cancer with stories about survivors and their families, clinical trials, and a Helpline at **(877) 573-9971** for those with questions.

I hope you have enjoyed this book and find it informative and inspirational. I also hope that you take the time and leave a review on my Amazon page!

Feel free to contact me on my Facebook page or by email. I am always happy to hear from readers!

Sarah Burton

9 781712 546437